The Obesity Epidemic

A Comprehensive Guide to Understanding, Treating and Preventing Obesity

Daniel I. Riggs

Table of content

1. INTRODUCTION

Obesity has become one of the most serious public health challenges of our time. It is a complex, multifaceted condition that affects people from all walks of life and all ages, genders, ethnicities, and socioeconomic backgrounds. This book will explore the causes and consequences of this epidemic in depth; examining how it impacts individuals and communities on a physical, mental, social, economic, and environmental level. We will look at how obesity can be addressed through lifestyle changes as well as medical interventions such as bariatric surgery. The aim is to provide readers with an understanding of this growing problem so they can make informed decisions about their health or that of loved ones.

This book will be a comprehensive guide to the obesity epidemic, exploring its causes and effects to improve public health. Through research and personal stories, we will delve into the complex nature of this condition to develop strategies for prevention, management, and treatment. With this knowledge, readers can take steps to protect themselves from the dangers of being overweight and obese while also learning how to support those around them. It is time to take action and address the obesity epidemic. This book will help readers do just that, providing an in-depth look at this pressing issue and offering practical solutions for improving public health. So, let's get started.

The obesity epidemic is one of the most pressing public health issues facing our society today. Its effects are far-reaching, ranging from increased risk of chronic illness to social and economic disadvantages. The World Health Organization estimates that more than 1.9 billion adults worldwide were overweight or obese in 2016, with 39% of adults aged 18 years and over classified as overweight and 13% classified as obese. In the United States alone, it is estimated that nearly 40 percent of adults are obese while 17 percent are severely so. This alarming rate has serious implications for our nation's physical and mental health as well as its economy; therefore, it is essential to recognize this issue for what it truly is: a complex problem requiring comprehensive solutions across multiple sectors.

1. Definition of Obesity

Obesity is a medical condition in which an individual has a body mass index (BMI) of 30 or higher. BMI is a measure of one's weight relative to their height, calculated by dividing the person's weight in kilograms by their squared height in meters (kg/m2). Being obese means having too much fat in your body, and this can lead to serious health problems such as type 2 diabetes, heart disease, stroke, and certain types of cancer. Obesity can also cause psychological issues such as depression and low self-esteem. People who are considered obese may need help from doctors and dietitians to develop healthy eating habits and exercise routines that will help them lose weight safely. Obesity is measured by BMI, but it can also be assessed by measuring the waist circumference of a person. Waist circumference measures how much fat is stored around the abdominal area and is used to identify people who are at higher risk for health problems due to their excess weight. People with a waist circumference greater than 40 inches (102 cm) for men or 35 inches (88 cm) for women are considered obese. The causes of obesity are complex and include both genetic and environmental factors. Eating an unhealthy diet, lack of physical activity, certain medications, medical conditions such as hypothyroidism or Cushing's syndrome, and genetics can all contribute to weight gain. In addition, people who have difficulty controlling their emotions may use food to cope with stress or other negative feelings.

II. Causes of Obesity

1. Unhealthy Diet: Eating too much high-fat, calorie-dense foods can lead to weight gain and obesity.
2. Lack of Physical Activity: Not engaging in physical activity regularly can contribute to weight gain and obesity over time.
3. Genetics: Having a family history of obesity increases the risk of developing it oneself since certain genes may affect metabolism or appetite

control in some people, leading to an increased tendency toward unhealthy eating habits or overeating.

4. Medications: Certain medications such as steroids, antidepressants, or antipsychotics can cause patients to gain weight due to their effects on hormones or metabolism regulation systems in the body that regulate food intake and energy expenditure levels.

5. Age: As people age, their metabolism slows down and they often become less active, leading to weight gain.

6. Stress: When a person is feeling stressed or anxious, they may turn to food for comfort which can lead to overeating and weight gain over time.

7. Lack of Sleep: People who don't get enough sleep can be at risk for developing obesity since lack of sleep disrupts hormones that control appetite and energy levels in the body.

8. Pregnancy: During pregnancy, women tend to gain weight as their bodies change to accommodate the growing baby.

9. Social and Economic Factors: People of lower socioeconomic status may be more likely to experience obesity due to limited access to healthy foods, lack of time or resources for physical activity, or exposure to higher levels of stress.

l Health Risks associated with obesity

Obesity is a major public health issue that can lead to numerous adverse physical and mental health risks. The most common physical health risks associated with obesity include:

1. Cardiovascular Disease (CVD): Obesity increases the risk of developing CVD, including coronary heart disease, stroke, peripheral artery disease, and congestive heart failure. This increased risk is due to factors such as high blood pressure and cholesterol levels or an increase in inflammation markers related to fat tissue deposits throughout the body.

2. Type 2 Diabetes: Excess weight increases insulin resistance which leads to type 2 diabetes; this form of diabetes has been linked with other chronic conditions such as kidney damage and eye problems like glaucoma or cataracts.

3. Certain Cancers: Excess weight has been linked to an increased risk of certain cancers, including breast cancer, colon cancer, endometrial cancer, kidney cancer, and gallbladder cancer.

4. Musculoskeletal Disorders: Excessive body fat can put added strain on the bones and joints leading to conditions such as osteoarthritis or low back pain. It can also lead to musculoskeletal injuries due to weakened muscles or tendons that are unable to cope with the extra weight being carried around in the body.

5. Metabolic Syndrome: This is a cluster of metabolic abnormalities that includes high blood pressure, high cholesterol levels, insulin resistance (leading to type 2 diabetes), and abdominal obesity.

6. Sleep Apnea: Obese individuals have a higher risk of developing sleep apnea, a condition in which breathing stops and starts during sleep due to an obstruction of the airway. This can lead to daytime fatigue and poor concentration,

as well as an increased risk of heart attack or stroke.

7. Psychological Issues: Obesity is associated with depression, anxiety, low self-esteem, and body image issues; these issues may be caused by the social stigma associated with being obese or simply due to the physical limitations that come along with excess weight.

In addition to the physical health risks associated with obesity, it can also lead to economic consequences such as increased healthcare costs, decreased productivity, and lost wages due to illness.

2. Diagnosing and Treating Obesity

Diagnosing obesity involves assessing a person's body mass index (BMI), which is calculated using height and weight. A BMI of 30 or higher indicates that someone is obese, while a BMI between 25 and 29.9 indicates that they are overweight. Other factors, such as waist circumference and risk for health problems related to being overweight or obese, may also be considered when diagnosing obesity.

In addition to measuring BMI, doctors will typically take into account other factors when diagnosing obesity. These include a family history of obesity-related conditions; lifestyle habits such as diet and physical activity level; any medical conditions that may contribute to excess weight gain; medications the patient is taking; sleep quality; mental health status; and overall health status.

If a person is found to be obese, the doctor may recommend lifestyle changes such as increasing physical activity and eating healthier foods. They may also refer the patient to a registered dietitian for nutrition counseling or suggest weight-loss medications or surgery if needed. Regular follow-up visits with the doctor are important for monitoring progress and adjusting treatment plans accordingly.

Overall, diagnosing obesity involves assessing a person's BMI and other factors to determine their risk for health problems related to being overweight or obese. Lifestyle changes and medical interventions may then be recommended if needed to help the patient reach a healthy weight.

- Treating Obesity

Treating obesity requires long-term changes in diet and physical activity habits as well as lifestyle modifications such as stress management. The first step in treating obesity is to identify any underlying causes of the condition such as hormonal imbalances or certain medications. If these are identified, they should be addressed with appropriate treatment before beginning any other interventions. Once underlying causes are ruled out or treated if applicable, lifestyle modifications should begin to help improve diet and physical activity habits.

This may involve seeing a dietitian develop an individualized meal plan that is tailored to the patient's needs and preferences as well as incorporating regular physical activity into their daily routine. It is also important for patients to be mindful of their eating patterns, such as when they eat, how much they eat, and what types of foods they are eating. In addition to lifestyle modifications, medications or weight-loss surgery can be considered in those with severe obesity who have not been able to achieve significant weight loss through lifestyle changes alone.

Medications can help reduce appetite or increase metabolism while surgical options such as gastric bypass or laparoscopic banding can alter gastrointestinal anatomy to limit food intake and promote weight loss. In addition to medical interventions, psychological and behavioral therapies can be used to help patients with obesity develop healthier eating and physical activity habits as well as improve their body image and self-esteem. These types of therapies can also help address any underlying psychological issues such as depression or anxiety that may be contributing to the condition. Finally, those with obesity need to receive ongoing support from family members, friends, healthcare providers, and other members of the community to ensure long-term success in managing the condition.

I. Screening for Obese Individuals

Screening in obese individuals is a process used to identify people who are at risk for developing health problems related to their weight. Screening typically involves assessing the individual's body mass index (BMI) and other factors such as waist circumference, blood pressure, cholesterol levels, and glucose levels. If any of these measurements are above normal ranges, then further testing may be recommended. For example, an abdominal ultrasound or CT scan can be performed to assess for fatty liver disease or gallstones; an echocardiogram can be done to evaluate heart function, and a fasting glucose test can be taken to check for diabetes. Additionally, lifestyle changes such as diet modification and increased physical activity should also be considered when screening obese individuals.

Screening for obesity-related health problems is important because many of these conditions can be managed or prevented if identified early. For example, lifestyle modifications such as diet and exercise can help reduce the risk of developing diabetes, heart disease, stroke, high blood pressure, and other chronic illnesses. Additionally, regular screenings can help identify individuals who may need more intensive interventions such as bariatric surgery or medication. Screening can also help to motivate individuals to make lifestyle changes that will improve their health and reduce the risk of developing obesity-related health problems in the future.

Overall, screening obese individuals is an important step to identify those at risk for developing chronic health problems. Regular screenings can help detect conditions early and allow for appropriate interventions to be put into place. Lifestyle modifications are also recommended as part of the screening process since these changes can reduce the risk of developing obesity-related illnesses over time.

II. Treatment Options For Obese Patients

Treatment options for obese patients depend on the severity of their obesity, as well as any underlying medical conditions they may have.

1. Lifestyle Changes: Making changes to lifestyle and diet is often the first step in treating obesity. This includes increasing physical activity, reducing calorie intake, eating healthier foods (such as fruits, vegetables, and whole grains), limiting portion sizes, avoiding sugary drinks or snacks high in fat/sugar content, and managing stress levels. It is important to create a plan that works for each patient based on their goals and preferences.

2. Medications: For some patients with severe obesity who are unable to lose weight through lifestyle modifications alone, medications can be prescribed by a doctor. These medications can help reduce appetite, increase feelings of fullness, or block fat absorption in the body.

Some common medications used to treat obesity include Orlistat (Xenical), Liraglutide (Saxenda), Phentermine/Topiramate (Qsymia), and Bupropion/Naltrexone (Contrave).

3. Surgery: In cases where lifestyle changes and medications are not enough to achieve desired weight loss results, surgery may be an option. Bariatric surgeries such as gastric bypass or sleeve gastrectomy can help people lose large amounts of weight by making changes to the digestive system that limit food intake and cause malabsorption of nutrients.

4. Alternative Treatments: In addition to the above treatments, there are also a variety of alternative therapies that can help people with obesity. These include cognitive-behavioral therapy (CBT), motivational interviewing, and hypnosis. Other treatments such as acupuncture, yoga, massage therapy, or herbal supplements may also be beneficial for some patients. No matter which treatment option is chosen, it is important to remember that long-term success in treating obesity requires commitment and dedication from both patient and doctor alike.

With the right approach and support system in place, individuals can achieve their desired weight loss goals while improving overall health and well-being.

III. Lifestyle Changes for weight loss and maintenance

Lifestyle changes for weight loss and maintenance involve making permanent alterations to one's diet and exercise habits. These changes should be tailored to the individual to ensure that they are achievable, sustainable, and effective.

When it comes to diet, a healthy eating plan should focus on nutritious foods such as fruits, vegetables, whole grains, lean proteins, low-fat dairy products, nuts, and seeds. It is important to limit processed foods high in sugar or salt content as well as saturated fat or trans fats. Calorie counting can also be helpful for some individuals who want more control over their food intake; however, this approach may not work for everyone.

Physical activity is also an essential part of any successful weight loss plan. It is recommended to get at least 150 minutes of moderate-intensity or 75 minutes of vigorous-intensity exercise per week to maintain a healthy weight. This can include activities such as walking, running, cycling, swimming, and strength training.

Other lifestyle changes that may help with weight loss and maintenance are getting adequate sleep each night (7-9 hours for adults), reducing stress levels through relaxation techniques such as yoga or meditation, limiting alcohol intake, and engaging in supportive relationships with friends and family members who can help keep you accountable on your journey towards a healthier lifestyle.

These lifestyle changes should be implemented gradually and with guidance from a healthcare professional to ensure the best outcomes. With patience, dedication, and support you can achieve your goals of weight loss and maintenance.

3. Preventing the Development of Obesity in Children & Adults

Preventing the development of obesity in children and adults requires a multi-faceted approach. There are both lifestyle changes that individuals can make as well as strategies to be implemented at the community level.

At an individual level, one of the most important steps is to ensure that healthy eating habits are established early on. This includes providing children with nutritious meals and snacks and limiting access to unhealthy foods such as those high in sugar or fat. It's also important for families to model healthy behaviors by engaging in regular physical activity together and avoiding sedentary activities like watching TV or playing video games for long periods.

In terms of physical activity, both adults and children alike need to get at least 30 minutes of exercise most days of the week, if not every day. This can include activities like walking, running, biking, swimming, or playing sports.

At a community level, there are several strategies that can be implemented to reduce obesity rates. These include providing access to affordable healthy food options and increasing the availability of public parks and recreational facilities for physical activity. Additionally, educational campaigns aimed at promoting healthy eating habits and physical activity should be encouraged in schools as well as in the media.

Overall, preventing the development of obesity requires both individual-level lifestyle changes as well as larger-scale interventions implemented at the community level. By making these changes we can help ensure that individuals remain healthy throughout their lives and reduce overall healthcare costs.

I. Nutrition Education Programs & Physical Activity Promotion

Nutrition education programs are designed to teach people about the importance of making healthy food choices and how to make those choices. These programs may be offered through schools, community organizations, healthcare providers, or other sources. They can include classroom activities as well as more interactive experiences such as cooking classes and grocery store tours. The goal is for participants to learn about nutrition facts, develop skills for selecting nutritious foods, and become aware of their eating habits to make informed decisions that support their overall health and well-being.

Physical activity promotion is an important part of a comprehensive approach to good health. It involves encouraging individuals and communities to be physically active by providing access to safe places for physical activity, offering incentives or rewards for being active, and providing education about the benefits of physical activity. It also includes creating policies and systems that make it easier for people to be physically active, such as providing bike-friendly routes or allowing employees to work remotely. Physical activity promotion is an important part of a comprehensive health strategy because regular physical activity can help reduce the risk of chronic diseases, improve overall mental and physical health, and promote healthy weight management.

In summary, nutrition education programs and physical activity promotion are two important strategies for promoting a healthy lifestyle. They both involve providing information, resources, and incentives to help people make informed decisions that support their overall health and well-being.

I. School-Based Interventions to Promote Healthy Eating Habits

School-based interventions are designed to promote healthy eating habits among students by providing them with the knowledge, skills, and resources needed to make healthy choices. These interventions typically include nutrition education, physical activity promotion, and changes to school food environments.

Nutrition Education: Nutrition education is an important part of any school-based intervention promoting healthy eating habits. It can involve teaching students about the importance of a balanced diet and how different foods impact their health. This type of education should be tailored to meet the needs of each age group and provide information that is relevant to their daily lives. Additionally, it should be provided in multiple formats (e.g., lectures, posters) so that all students have access to this information regardless of learning style or preferred method of instruction. Physical Activity Promotion: Physical activity is an important component of a healthy lifestyle and should be promoted in schools as part of any intervention. This can involve providing students with opportunities to participate in physical activities during school hours (e.g., recess, PE classes) or after-school programs that encourage physical activity through sports, games, and other activities. Additionally, promoting active transportation (e.g., walking or biking to school) can help make physical activity a part of the daily routine for students.

Changes to School Food Environments: In addition to nutrition education and physical activity promotion, interventions should also focus on making changes to the food environment within schools so that healthier options are available and accessible for students. This can include providing healthier food choices in school cafeterias, snack bars, and vending machines; increasing access to fresh fruits and vegetables; reducing the availability of unhealthy snacks such as candy and chips; and encouraging students to bring healthy lunches from home.

These are just a few examples of strategies that can be used as part of school-based interventions to promote healthy eating habits among students. By implementing these strategies, schools can help create an environment where it is easier for students to make healthier choices when it comes to their diet.

III. Workplace Interventions to Promote Healthy Eating & Exercise

Workplace Intervention to promote healthy Eating and Exercise Workplace interventions to promote healthy eating and exercise involve making changes in the workplace environment that encourage employees to make healthier choices. This includes providing access to healthy food options, offering incentives for physical activity, and creating a culture of health through education and communication strategies.

1 Healthy Food Options: Providing access to nutritious foods is an important part of promoting healthy eating at work. This can include offering fresh fruits and vegetables as snacks or meals during meetings, stocking vending machines with healthier snack options such as nuts or granola bars instead of candy or chips, providing free water dispensers throughout the office space, and ensuring there are adequate nutrition labels on all food items available for purchase in cafeterias or from vending machines.

2 Incentives for Physical Activity: Offering incentives or rewards for physical activity can be an effective way to motivate employees to stay active. This could include offering discounted gym memberships, providing access to on-site fitness centers, organizing team sports activities during lunch breaks or after work hours, and offering subsidized classes such as yoga or Zumba.

3 Education and Communication Strategies: Educating employees about the benefits of healthy eating and exercise is essential in promoting a culture of health in the workplace. Companies should provide information on nutrition guidelines, healthy food choices, how to incorporate physical activity into daily routines, and tips for maintaining good mental health. Additionally, companies should create communication strategies that keep employees informed about available resources or programs related to healthy eating and physical activity.

Overall, workplace interventions to promote healthy eating and exercise can help create an environment that encourages employees to make better choices for their health. By providing access to nutritious foods, offering incentives for physical activity, and educating employees on the benefits of a healthy lifestyle, companies can create a culture of health in the workplace.

4. Meal Planning for Obesity Patients

Meal planning for obesity patients is an important step in helping individuals reach their weight loss goals. A healthy diet and regular exercise are key components of a successful weight loss plan, so it's essential to create an eating plan that meets the individual's needs while also promoting overall health. The first step in meal planning for obese patients is to determine what types of foods they should be eating daily. This includes lean proteins such as fish, skinless poultry, eggs, and tofu; complex carbohydrates like whole grains, beans, and legumes; non-starchy vegetables such as leafy greens, broccoli, cauliflower, peppers, and onions; low-fat dairy products like yogurt or cottage cheese; fruits; and healthy fats like olive oil, nuts, and avocado. It's important to make sure that the diet is balanced with all of these food groups to ensure adequate nutrition. The next step is to create a meal plan that incorporates these foods into daily meals and snacks. This should include three main meals (breakfast, lunch, and dinner) as well as two or three smaller snacks throughout the day. For each meal or snack, aim for at least one serving from each food group listed above. To help keep calories under control, pay attention to portion sizes; using measuring cups can be helpful for this task. Finally, it's important to remember that healthy eating isn't just about avoiding unhealthy foods

## I.	7-day meal plan For Obese Patient

Day 1:

Breakfast: Oatmeal with Fresh Berries

Ingredients: -1 cup rolled oats -2 cups water or almond milk -½ teaspoon ground cinnamon (optional) -1/3 cup fresh berries of your choice (blueberries, strawberries, raspberries etc.)

Instructions: Bring the water or almond milk to a boil in a small pot over medium heat. Add the oats and decrease the intensity to low. Simmer for 4 minutes stirring occasionally. Remove from heat and stir in the cinnamon if desired. Divide oatmeal among two bowls and top each bowl with half of the fresh berries before serving.

Lunch: Quinoa Salad with Chickpeas

Ingredients: -1 cup quinoa, cooked according to package instructions -1 can chickpeas (15 ounces), drained and rinsed -1/2 cup diced red onion -3 tablespoons fresh lemon juice -2 tablespoons extra virgin olive oil

Instructions: In a large bowl, combine the cooked quinoa, chickpeas, red onion and lemon juice. Drizzle with olive oil and stir until all of the ingredients are evenly distributed. Serve at room temperature or chilled.

Dinner: Grilled Chicken with Roasted Vegetables

Ingredients: -4 boneless skinless chicken breasts -2 teaspoons garlic powder -2 teaspoons dried oregano -2 tablespoons olive oil -1 red bell pepper, diced -one green bell pepper, diced -one zucchini, sliced into rounds

Instructions: Preheat the oven to four hundred degrees Fahrenheit. Place the chicken breasts on a baking sheet and season with garlic powder and oregano. Drizzle with olive oil and bake for

20 minutes or until cooked through. Meanwhile, place the vegetables in a large bowl and toss with 2 teaspoons of olive oil. Spread onto a separate baking sheet and roast for 15 minutes or until tender. Serve grilled chicken topped with roasted vegetables.

Day 2:

Breakfast: Avocado Toast with Egg

Ingredients: -2 slices whole-grain bread -1 ripe avocado, pitted and mashed -2 eggs, fried or poached -Salt and pepper to taste

Instructions: Toast the slices of bread in a toaster. Spread the pounded avocado onto each cut of toast. Top with a fried or poached egg and season with salt and pepper before serving.

Lunch: Turkey Wrap with Spinach

Ingredients: -4 ounces sliced turkey breast deli meat -2 whole wheat tortillas -2 cups baby spinach leaves -½ cup plain Greek yogurt

Instructions: Lay out two tortillas on a work surface. Divide the turkey among them, laying it in an even layer over one half of each tortilla. Top with spinach and spread the Greek yogurt over the turkey. Roll up tightly and cut in half before serving.

Dinner: Baked Salmon with Asparagus

Ingredients: -4 (4 ounce) salmon fillets -1 tablespoon olive oil -2 cloves garlic, minced -1 lemon, sliced into rounds -1 pound asparagus spears, trimmed

Instructions: Preheat oven to 400 degrees Fahrenheit. Place salmon fillets on a baking sheet lined with parchment paper or aluminum foil and brush lightly with olive oil on both sides. Sprinkle garlic over top of the fish and lay lemon slices in an even layer around it. Arrange asparagus spears around the salmon. Heat for 15 minutes or until the fish is cooked through and the asparagus is delicate.

Day 3:

Breakfast: Greek Yogurt Parfait with Berries

Ingredients: -1 cup plain Greek yogurt -¼ cup granola of your choice -½ cup fresh berries (strawberries, blueberries, raspberries etc.)

Instructions: Layer the ingredients in a bowl beginning with Greek yogurt, followed by granola and topped off with fresh berries. Enjoy cold!

Lunch: Tuna Salad Sandwich on Whole Grain Bread

Ingredients: -2 cans tuna packed in water, drained and flaked -¼ cup diced red onion -2 tablespoons chopped fresh parsley -3 tablespoons mayonnaise -4 slices whole grain bread

Instructions: In a medium bowl, combine tuna, red onion, parsley and mayonnaise. Spread an even layer of the mixture over two slices of bread before topping with the remaining two. Cut in half and serve.

Dinner: Baked Sweet Potato Fries with Turkey Burgers

Ingredients: -1 pound lean ground turkey -¼ cup diced onion -1 teaspoon garlic powder -4 sweet potatoes, cut into thin strips -2 tablespoons olive oil

Instructions: Preheat oven to 425 degrees Fahrenheit. Line a baking sheet with material paper or aluminum foil. In a medium bowl, combine ground turkey, onion and garlic powder. Form into four patties and place on the prepared baking sheet. Toss sweet potato strips with olive oil in a separate bowl before spreading in an even layer around the burgers on the baking sheet. Bake for 25 minutes or until burgers are cooked through and sweet potatoes are golden brown.

Day 4

Breakfast: Fruit Smoothie

Ingredients: -1 banana -½ cup frozen strawberries -¼ cup plain Greek yogurt -1 tablespoon honey -¾ cup almond milk (or any other type of milk)

Instructions: Preheat a grill or a grill container to medium-high intensity. Grill the vegetables until they are softly burned and delicate. Enjoy cold!

Lunch: Grilled Vegetable and Hummus Wrap

Ingredients: -2 whole wheat tortillas -1 cup cooked vegetables of your choice (bell peppers, zucchini, eggplant etc.) -½ cup hummus of your choice

Instructions: Preheat the grill or grill pan to medium-high intensity. Grill the vegetables until they are daintily roasted and delicate. Spread an even layer of hummus over each tortilla before adding grilled vegetables down the center. Roll up tightly and cut in half before serving.

Dinner: Baked Salmon Cakes with Quinoa

Ingredients: -2 (4 ounce) salmon fillets -¼ cup diced red onion -2 tablespoons chopped fresh parsley -1 cup cooked quinoa -2 tablespoons olive oil

Instructions: Preheat oven to 400 degrees Fahrenheit. Place salmon fillets in a baking dish and sprinkle with red onion and parsley. Heat for 15 minutes or until fish is cooked through delicate. Flake the salmon into a large bowl and add the cooked quinoa, stirring to combine. Form mixture into four patties and brush both sides lightly with olive oil before transferring to a parchment paper lined baking sheet. Heat for 10 minutes or until golden brown on each side.

Day 5

Breakfast: Overnight Oats with Apples

Ingredients: -1 cup rolled oats -2 cups almond milk (or any other type of milk) -½ teaspoon ground cinnamon (optional) -1 apple, diced

Instructions: Place oats and almond milk in a mason jar or other container with a lid. Stir to combine and add the cinnamon if desired. Seal the lid tightly and shake to mix everything together. Refrigerate overnight before stirring in the diced apples before serving cold or at room temperature.

Lunch: Turkey Lettuce Wraps with Avocado

Ingredients: -4 ounces sliced turkey breast deli meat -2 large lettuce leaves -1 ripe avocado, pitted and mashed -2 tablespoons plain Greek yogurt

Instructions: Divide turkey among two lettuce leaves, laying it in an even layer over one half of each leaf Spread the mashed avocado over the turkey and top with a dollop of Greek yogurt. Fold in half and enjoy!

Dinner: Baked Cod with Roasted Vegetables

Ingredients: -4 (4 ounce) cod fillets -1 tablespoon olive oil -2 cloves garlic, minced -1 red pepper, diced -1 zucchini, sliced into rounds -Salt and pepper to taste

Instructions: Preheat oven to Four hundred degrees Fahrenheit Place cod fillets on a baking sheet lined with parchment paper or aluminum foil and brush lightly with olive oil on both sides. Sprinkle garlic over top of the fish before arranging vegetables around it. Season everything lightly with salt and pepper before baking for 15 minutes or until fish is cooked through and vegetables are tender.

Day 6

Breakfast: Egg White Omelet with Spinach

Ingredients: -4 egg whites -½ cup baby spinach leaves -¼ cup diced red pepper -2 tablespoons reduced fat shredded cheese of your choice (optional)

Instructions: Heat a small nonstick skillet over medium heat. Add the egg whites and cook for 1 minute before stirring in the spinach, red pepper and cheese if desired. Cook for an additional 2-3 minutes, stirring occasionally, until eggs are cooked through. Serve warm!

Lunch: Avocado Chicken Salad Sandwich on Whole Grain Bread

Ingredients: -1 cup cooked chicken breast -1 ripe avocado, pitted and mashed -2 tablespoons plain Greek yogurt -4 slices whole grain bread

Instructions: In a medium bowl, combine cooked chicken, mashed avocado and Greek yogurt. Spread an even layer of the mixture over two slices of bread before topping with the remaining two. Cut in half and serve.

Dinner: Baked Sweet Potato Fries with Grilled Chicken Breasts

Ingredients: -4 boneless skinless chicken breasts -2 teaspoons garlic powder -2 teaspoons dried oregano -4 sweet potatoes, cut into thin strips -3 tablespoons olive oil

Instructions: Preheat oven to 425 degrees Fahrenheit. Line a baking sheet with material paper or aluminum foil. Place chicken breasts on a separate baking sheet and season with garlic powder and oregano. Drizzle with 2 tablespoons of olive oil before transferring to the oven. Toss sweet potato strips with remaining tablespoon of olive oil in a large bowl before spreading in an even layer around the chicken on the baking sheet. Bake for 25 minutes or until chicken is cooked through and sweet potatoes are golden brown.

Day 7
Breakfast: Banana Oat Pancakes
Ingredients: -1 ripe banana, mashed -2 eggs -½ cup rolled oats -¼ teaspoon ground cinnamon (optional)
Instructions: In a medium bowl, mash the banana until smooth. Put the eggs and mix into a single unit until consolidated. Stir in the oats and cinnamon if desired. Heat a large nonstick skillet over medium heat and lightly grease with oil or cooking spray. Drop the batter by ¼ cupfuls onto the preheated skillet, spreading into circles about 4 inches wide. Cook for 2-3 minutes before flipping to cook on the other side for an additional 1-2 minutes until golden brown. Serve warm with fresh fruit of your choosing!
Lunch: Greek Salad with Quinoa
Ingredients: -1 cup cooked quinoa -2 cups chopped romaine lettuce -½ cup diced red onion -¼ cup feta cheese crumbles -3 tablespoons extra virgin olive oil
Instructions: In a large bowl, combine cooked quinoa , lettuce, red onion and feta cheese. Drizzle with olive oil and stir until all of the

ingredients are evenly distributed. Serve chilled or at room temperature.

Dinner: Baked Salmon with Asparagus

Ingredients: -4 (4 ounce) salmon fillets -1 tablespoon olive oil -2 cloves garlic, minced -1 lemon, sliced into rounds -1 pound asparagus spears, trimmed

Instructions: Preheat oven to 400 degrees Fahrenheit. Place salmon fillets on a baking sheet lined with parchment paper or aluminum foil and brush lightly with olive oil on both sides. Sprinkle garlic over top of the fish and lay lemon slices in an even layer around it. Arrange asparagus spears around the salmon. Heat for 15 minutes or until the fish is cooked through and the asparagus is delicate.

5. Conclusion

The obesity epidemic is an ever-growing problem, but it can be solved if we take the right steps. We need to bring awareness to this issue and ensure that people have access to healthy foods and physical activities. We also need better education about nutrition, exercise, and lifestyle choices so that people can make informed decisions about their health. With these efforts in place, we can help reduce the prevalence of obesity across all ages and ultimately create a healthier society for everyone.

This book has explored the complexity of the obesity epidemic, from its causes to its potential solutions. We now have a better understanding of how this problem affects our society and what steps we can take to address it. With continued focus and dedication to healthy living, we can make progress in tackling this pressing issue.

It is up to us to make the changes necessary for a healthier future. We must take action now and be part of the solution, not the problem. With this in mind, let us all work together towards creating a world free from obesity.

www.ingramcontent.com/pod-product-compliance
Lightning Source LLC
Chambersburg PA
CBHW051717250726
48653CB00007B/3073